Anne Duval

Apple Cider Vinegar Cure

A Complete Guide to Discover the Apple Cider Vinegar Benefits. Recipes & Remedies to Naturally cure your Body

Table of Contents

Apple Cider Vinegar Cure

Apple cider vinegar is a product of fermentation of apple juice. It would seem that nothing extraordinary, but in fact, its advantages are immeasurable. Healthy properties were well known long before our time. Hippocrates prescribed it as a disinfectant. The Greeks and Romans drank a drink. Columbus took him to the sails. The Samurai drank it with force, as did the Babylonians and Caesar's soldiers.

In modern times, many authors claimed to use it for different purposes. Some wrote testimonies about how they lowered cholesterol, normalized weight and increased energy in their patients and themselves. If as a reader you find one of these interesting, do not hesitate to conduct further research.

Before we begin, I would like to emphasize that the substance we are discussing here is not something that you can find on the shelf of an ordinary supermarket. Most of the vinegar sold in Chains is too diluted to have many health-promoting qualities. You want organic vinegar, raw and undiluted. This type of apple cider vinegar is usually found in healthy food stores. A good kind of apple cider vinegar will contain a lot of vitamins, organic acids, minerals, pectin and enzymes.

That's what this amazing substance can do for athletes.

Taken inside:

It replaces minerals lost by sweat and used for metabolic functions. Muscle contraction and relaxation cycle require a basic four minerals (magnesium, sodium, potassium and calcium), which are all found in the apple vinegar. LCA also contributes to the elimination of lactic acid, thereby speeding up recovery.

Applied externally:

Prevents swelling associated with strains, sprains, bruises and aching muscles.

Start with a few drops per cup of water.

Many people like the taste of this drink. If not, try adding a teaspoon of honey to the drink, as recommended by the famous Bragg Family. In case you are allergic to beekeeping products, try using dehydrated, raw and organic sugar cane instead of honey. You may be pleasantly surprised by the effect of this drink on your Sports Performance.

Be careful - if you think you have yeast or fungus infestation, avoid using this drink until the problem is solved.

To use apple cider vinegar outside, it is enough to soak the cloth in vinegar and apply to the target area. Cover with a plastic wrap or dry cloth. Personally, I have heard and experienced several cases where a potentially dangerous edema was greatly minimized when you use the apple cider vinegar. This substance may not be able to magically reverse the damage, but it can significantly slow down the swelling and accelerate recovery.

As always, be sure to see your health care provider as soon as possible.

As the Old English proverb says: "Eat an apple before going to bed, will force the doctor to beg for his bread"

The Unique Wonders of Apple Cider Vinegar

Apple cider vinegar (ACV) is one of the most useful and comprehensive home remedies. This is invaluable as a general health tonic at 1 teaspoon per day. Soaking the cotton swabs in apple cider vinegar and placing the wart begins a quick process of killing the wart to the roots. Wrapping a cotton swab in tape overnight and repeating it anywhere in 2-4 nights will often lead to the death of the wart. Apple cider vinegar also kills worm and Tinea.

Other diseases that apple cider vinegar is known to cure are throat pain, hypercholesterolemia, acne, allergies, muscle fatigue, immune system disorders, weight loss, constipation, arthritis, gout, bladder stones, bad breath, cellulite and urinary tract infections.

Apple cider vinegar contains natural bacterial agents, as well as many minerals and elements such as potassium, calcium, magnesium, phosphorus, chlorine, sodium, sulfur, copper, iron and Silicon.

The natural method of making apple cider vinegar is the crushing of fresh apples (preferably organic) and their ripening in wooden barrels. This increases the quality of the natural process of Apple fermentation. It is important to note that it is completely different from the refined vinegar that is found mainly in supermarkets. Natural vinegar has enzymes and minerals that other too processed vinegar may not have.

As already mentioned, any AKV is better than anyone, and the ACV Super Market can be the most accessible and cheapest for many people. In this case, I suggest that whatever type of stroke you are able to get is still going to be fantastic for your health.

The Miracles of Apple Cider Vinegar

Have you ever wondered what miracle cures are found in your house for various diseases? The next time you're in the store, consider buying a bottle of apple cider vinegar. You can simply be surprised at how versatile and beneficial this cheap vinegar is. Apple cider vinegar contains various vitamins and minerals and has many health benefits.

Before the dawn of our calendar, it was reported that Hippocrates, the "father of Medicine", used it for his patients. Apple cider vinegar is made from fermentation of fresh and ripe apples. It contains vitamins like beta-carotene and pectin and mineral substances such as calcium, magnesium, phosphorus, potassium and iron. It can be used as part of many recipes including salad dressing, marinade, meat tenderizer and pickling. In search of the best apple cider vinegar look for natural and organic varieties, which are dark and turbid, because of the bright and sparkling types have very low nutritional value. It can be consumed every morning, adding two teaspoons to 8-12oz. a glass of water, with organic honey and lemon juice if its taste is too strong for its acidity. Apple cider vinegar is loaded with health benefits, with the sample shown below:

- Reduce cholesterol and regulate blood pressure and blood sugar due to its pectin content. It'll help with diabetes.
- Fights bacterial, fungal and yeast information by regulating the body pH due to its content of malic and acetic acid.
- It can relieve joint pain and help with GOUT by dissolving the uric acid crystals, as well as help prevent kidney and bladder stones.
- Helps with hair loss, brittle nails and teeth due to its potassium content.
- Helps with weight loss by reducing fat.
- It helps with acne, other bad and body odor, due to its acid content, odor breakdown causing bacteria and reducing pH. gargle a tablespoon of apple cider vinegar with water for five to ten minutes.
- Removes foot odor by inserting the legs into the pan with the water and 1/3 cup of apple cider vinegar for 15 minutes a week.
- It helps with diarrhea, since the content of pectin covers the lining of the large intestine. Drink two tablespoons with a large glass of water three times a day.

- It can help with age machines, due to the sulfur content.
- Treat dandruff by destroying the fungus on the head and restoring the correct pH balance. Try to apply a mixture of half water and half apple cider vinegar directly to the scalp, allowing natural drying.
- It provides relief from sunburn. Moisten the canvas with apple cider vinegar and gently apply to sunburn. You can also put the affected part of the body in a bath of apple cider vinegar.
- Increases the immune system due to beta-carotene, which has
- Can help with sinusitis and rhinitis due to its potassium content
- It helps with sore throat. Gargle with a teaspoon of apple cider vinegar and eight ounces of warm water with lemon.

This can help with ear information, diluting the diluted solution of apple cider vinegar and sweeping the inner ear.

Many people decide to drink a diluted solution of apple cider vinegar and water every day for health benefits. Side effects are close to none, but may cause breakage of tooth enamel if consumed too often in undiluted condition. Just add water or a pinch of baking soda when consuming to avoid any deterioration of enamel. From increasing immunity to regulating blood sugar, apple cider vinegar is very versatile. A 2004 study in the American Diabetes Society entitled "vinegar improve sensitivity" insulin having a high carbohydrate meal in subjects with insulin resistance and type 2 diabetes" found that apple cider vinegar contains acetic acid which can slow down carbohydrate digestion, reducing glucose levels in the blood. Apple Cider vinegar is easy and safe to buy and use, and can be used as a wonderful alternative to help your health. It remains one of the most popular and inexpensive immediate health alternatives on the market today.

Apple Cider Vinegar as Treatment for Acid Reflux

We all know that apples can do miracles in our lives. A very useful Apple product is apple cider vinegar. This type of vinegar is very common in homes and is very effective in the treatment of acne, sinus infections, allergies, hypercholesterolemia, Candida, flu, contact dermatitis, chronic fatigue, gout, arthritis, sore throat, and, most importantly, acid reflux.

Yeah, you read it right. If you are one of those people who suffer from reflux of acid, but do not know how to cure it, apple cider may be best for you answers. This is a natural way to treat and can cost less than antacids available on the pharmacy counter. However, do not expect that it will immediately treat reflux at once. Going for natural remedies can take time to actually see the effects or results. That's why patience is really very important here.

If you have enough patience, and I do not wish to go for manufacturers of drugs and opt for natural, recommended dose of apple cider should be 2 to 3 teaspoons in an eight-ounce glass of water before meals or whenever heartburn is known. You can repeat this three times a day, and if you are currently treating the disease, you may need a stronger mixture. Many people do not like the taste of this remedy. Some can also experience a sour or metallic taste and burning tongue. But if you really want to heal, you have to endure the consequences. The good thing is that no matter what brand you want to use, until it is made from cider, then everything will be fine. And it really does miracles!!!

The theory behind this natural remedy is acetic acid, which is found in vinegar helps to reduce acidity in the stomach because acetic acid is much lower than the hydrochloric acid. It is also believed that acetic acid with acetate salt can also help maintain and buffer gastric acid at PH 3.0. In this regard a milder acidic environment will be carried out and the stomach can effectively digest the food, causing less problems with the esophagus and lead to less heartburn.

Medicinal Uses of Apple Cider Vinegar

Apple cider vinegar has become a mark in the history of Medicine. Its use dates back to Babylonian times, but owes its new popularity around the world Hippocrates, who recognized his potential, and prescribed it as an antibiotic-especially for flu and other illnesses with flu-like symptoms.

Today, millions of people are still dependent on the available gift of nature. As regards the treatment of symptoms, clinically or scientifically proven or not, gaining the respect of the medicinal world, because it's all natural and organic, and it seems that a lot of people good and happy. As many would say, it won't hurt you, so try.

But what is this disease, apple cider vinegar? And besides, what theories surround its effectiveness?

At the top of the list, it can be locally said that apple cider vinegar heals acne. Vinegar itself is known as a good cleanser due to its acidity. The same principle can be used to cleanse the skin of oils that cause acne. A very weak mixture of water-based vinegar can be applied to the affected areas using cotton wool. This, followed by abundant rinsing with water, can be done daily, preferably before bedtime. In a few days, acne should be dried naturally and emptied with swelling and redness. As a bonus, hundreds of dollars of potential savings from expensive face care products.

Perhaps the most common disease is apple cider vinegar is known for the common cold, even cough until it comes to phlegm and swollen air passages. I repeat, a mixture of water based beverages, usually in combination with honey for taste can be taken up to three times a day during the lactation period. It is known that the mixture restores the acidity of the body, which significantly decreases in the fight against infection.

On another note, the same mixture, without honey, can be boiled by steam inhalation. It can more effectively clean the nostrils. As a bonus, People report that they will relieve their headaches even during the process.

Less well-known condition associated with apple cider vinegar arthritis, especially gouty arthritis or simply gout. It is believed that when consuming apple cider vinegar is produced the blood alkaline, which reduces the level of uric acid-the culprit in this particular form of arthritis. However, this treatment is usually taken at long intervals and is better known as a control mechanism. Some report that after the end of treatment, their symptoms continue to progress normally.

At this time, we listed diseases that are not categorical or similar, but still related to apple cider vinegar. This affects only the surface of real healing forces, for which this type of vinegar is known. There are many other remedies associated with this product, which only comes from your everyday apples. In part, it also shows us the unlimited resources with which mother nature has blessed, and it's just a piece of that cake.

Health Benefits of Apple Cider Vinegar

Apple cider vinegar cures many ailments. It's a pity that most people do not know. That's why I'm here to tell you the benefits of drinking apple cider vinegar.

Diseases such as arthritis, constipation, acne, gout, sore throat, hypertension, weight problems and a myriad of other health problems can be helped and even cured by drinking apple cider vinegar.

Why is it so special that it can be used as a remedy for these health problems and why is it better than other vinegar? It is the nutritional value that is in apple cider vinegar that makes it too much against various diseases.

This vinegar is made from chopped fresh apples, which are put in wooden barrels to allow natural fermentation. Natural apple cider vinegar should have a rich brown color. When you look into the light, you will see brown particles that look like cobwebs. This substance is called "Mother". As you get older, you will see more mothers piling up on the bottom of the bottle.

Natural apple cider vinegar has a strong smell, which is a good sign. In the "maternal substance" there is an abundance of healthy nutrients. Unfiltered natural apple cider vinegar showed strong health benefits.

Some of the nutrients that give it its healing powers are iron, copper, trace elements, phosphorus, silicon, essential amino acids, sulphur, magnesium, sodium, natural organic, fluoro organic, natural and many other powerful nutrients.

A nutrient that is loaded with apple cider vinegar, which is the key to youth, is potassium. Potassium helps to build and maintain young and healthy tissues. Potassium also helps to slow down the process of hardening and clogging, which can kill the cardiovascular system.

The vinegar you see on the shelves of supermarkets are all devoid of nutritional value, since these vinegars are distilled and pasteurized, which means that "mother" has been removed.

Most people use vinegar as a flavor and do not think of it as a nutritional drink. Vinegar producers do not intend to educate the public about the important health benefits of natural apple cider vinegar, because they are not aware of these benefits.

It's really sad because people lack a great flavor that adds to food the nutritional value it has for a product that has no nutritional value and can cause more harm than benefit.

Ordinary vinegar, which you can see on the shelves is distilled, pasteurized vinegar, people prefer it because they are not aware of what they actually consume.

If they were educated on apple cider vinegar, they would choose it rather than commercial vinegar.

People think that pure vinegar is healthy because it looks clean, but it only seems because it has been stripped of all its nutritional value. Eating these vinegars can harm your health. Commercial vinegar does not have vitamins, minerals or potassium that the body needs.

Don't let them discourage you from using it. The brown color with sediment on the bottom of the bottle does not look as good as the crystalline vinegar you see at the supermarket. The proof is not how it looks, but how it can change your health.

With all the great benefits it can offer, it makes sense to incorporate it into your daily health regimen. What you do not hurt, you can only strengthen and have shown that they can strengthen your health by providing you with the nutrients that your body needs.

Apple cider vinegar has many benefits for your health. It's no surprise, because Oprah, 20/20 and CBS, to name a few, are all excited about the apple cider vinegar and its benefits.

There are also many books written about apple cider vinegar describing how excellent it is for your health. The best-selling books on this topic include Patricia Bragg miracle Health system apple cider vinegar, Earl Mindell's amazing apple cider vinegar Cynthia holzapfel of is apple cider vinegar for weight loss and good health, and Dr. Karkar's apple cider vinegar remedies and treats.

Proponents believe that apple cider vinegar can cure or help with a myriad of diseases and health problems, such as arthritis, osteoporosis, high blood pressure, hypercholesterolemia, cancer, infection, indigestion, memory and aging. In addition, the most talked about the benefits of apple cider vinegar is apparently its help in weight loss.

Here are some of the main benefits of apple cider vinegar:

1. apple cider vinegar and weight loss

2. apple cider vinegar and acid reflux

3. apple cider vinegar and acne

4. apple cider vinegar and warts

5. apple cider vinegar and heartburn

6. apple cider vinegar and yeast infection

7. apple cider vinegar and arthritis

8. apple cider vinegar on the skin

9. apple cider vinegar and cholesterol

10. apple cider vinegar for hair

11. apple cider vinegar and blood pressure

12. apple cider vinegar for breast infection

13. apple cider vinegar and candida

14. apple cider vinegar and gout

15. apple cider vinegar and detoxification

16. apple cider vinegar and dandruff

17. apple cider vinegar and Gerd

18. apple cider vinegar and hair loss

19. apple cider vinegar and constipation

15. apple cider vinegar and diabetes

Apple cider vinegar is good for you. With many benefits, it's no wonder why many people talk about apple cider vinegar and what it can do for your health.

If you find the idea of drinking a full teaspoon of apple cider vinegar too difficult, taking apple cider vinegar pills can be a good alternative for you.

Does Apple Cider Vinegar Cure Acne

Will apple cider vinegar cure acne? Yes, cider is one of the best home remedies that you can use to remove pimples and acne spots. It is used easily, and there are no side effects when using this remedy for acne.

Vinegar is produced by fermentation of vegetables, fruits and cereals. Food molecules are decomposed with the help of yeast and bacteria. Sugars turn into alcohol, so fermentation turns alcohol into vinegar. In this book you will learn how to use apple cider vinegar to clarify the symptoms of acne.

Apple cider vinegar differs from ordinary vinegar. Vinegar is made from fermentation of crushed apples in wooden barrels. It contains more enzymes and minerals than other vinegars. This vinegar is loaded with calcium, potassium, copper, magnesium, phosphorus and iron. Apple cider contains antioxidants like vitamin a And C, beta-carotene and 3 different forms of vitamin B, and bioflavonoids etc...

So, apple cider vinegar heals acne? Here's how you can use cider to eliminate acne. There are three ways to use cider to treat acne. Use it as a tonic for the skin or to apply it directly on the affected area, or you can drink it as a health tonic, always works, that you want to use for the treatment of acne.

Before applying to pimples and pimples, always dilute apple cider vinegar with water. Mix 2 tablespoons of cider for 1 ounce of water. Use a cotton swab and soak it in a solution, and then soak it for acne. Leave the pimples for about 15 minutes to rinse. Do it two or three times a day, and your face will soon look better.

Cider will reduce infection and inflammation of acne. When you leave the cider for the night, when you wake up in the morning, your pimples and pimples begin to dry out. Do it several times a day, if you can.

If you use cider as a toner, you can adjust the pH balance of the skin and remove excess oil from the surface of the skin. Fill the sink and add a cup of vinegar and spray your face with water. Of course, do this after washing and drying the face. The solution kills bacteria and bacteria on the skin, so it is normal to do it several times a day.

Drinking apple cider vinegar as a health tonic is a great way to reduce further epidemics and help prevent further acne. Add 1 to 2 teaspoons of cider to a cup of warm water add a little honey to improve the taste and drink this mixture 3 times a day. Do not forget to rinse your mouth after drinking this tonic, because vinegar is very sour and could damage your teeth.

Use cider every day and you will see an improvement in acne condition and an improvement in skin clarity within a few days. Remember that natural home remedy and home remedies are not as strong as a commercial product you can use to treat acne.

Apple cider vinegar heals acne, clarifies the symptoms of acne on the skin, so if this is the medicine you are looking for, the answer is yes to the question. However, treating only the symptoms of acne is not a cure. If you really want to get rid of acne, you need to take steps to treat acne from the inside and outside.

What you need to remember with a home remedy is that it takes longer to remove the symptoms of acne than commercial treatments. However, the top side of home treatment is that it is inexpensive and that there are no harmful side effects when used.

Many today switch to natural home remedies in order to save money by purchasing those expensive skin solutions that they claim can cure acne but never fulfill their promises. There is a growing trend of awareness among the community to go for natural treatments and this is certainly bad news for the commercial skin markets.

There are a number of natural home remedies available. Among them, apple cider vinegar. You would probably read a lot of articles about the use of apple cider vinegar as a remedy for adult acne. Does it really work? How is that true? I hope this b can dispel some misconceptions about this home natural remedy, if any.

How to make apple cider vinegar?

Apple cider vinegar is obtained by fermentation of cider or cider made from crushed organic apples. FYI, fermentation is an act of conversion. Organic apples have bacteria and yeast on their skin. So, when they are crushed, you get a pure apple juice with a mixture of bacteria and yeast.

Then let it ripen for a while. During this process, sugar in cider spreads on yeast and bacteria that turn into alcohol. It is more of a fermentation process that eventually turns into vinegar after the second fermentation.

If you do not have the time or resources to create one at home, you can easily buy apple cider vinegar in any department store. First, be sure to get an organic LCA with labels that say " Mom's ideal acidity (pH) at a level of five to seven. This means that it is in raw and pure form characterized by a dark, turbid bacterial foam, similar to a canvas of brownish color.

Benefits of apple cider vinegar for your skin

ACV contains acids, one of which is alpha-hydroxyl acid, which was extracted directly from apples. These acids help dissolve oil and sebum, which clog the pores and eventually clog them. This will promote skin renewal.

It is known to treat pet allergies, food and environmental pollution, high cholesterol, influenza, chronic fatigue, breast infection, sore throat, arthritis and gout, to name a few.

However, its most popular advantage is associated with weight loss. ACV is known to break down fats and that the daily dose of apple cider vinegar in water helps keep blood pressure under control in just two weeks.

It also helps to adjust the pH of the skin by simply diluting it with two parts of water and spreading the mixture on the face with a cotton swab as a toner overnight and washing it until the morning. Know that dilute it with more water, while going on vacation on your skin for long hours.

It also helps to lighten age spots by rubbing ACV directly about twenty minutes a day, depending on their size. In addition, it also helps to cleanse the liver by removing accumulated toxins and recharging their effectiveness.

How is apple cider vinegar used for acne?

The use varies depending on the severity of acne. Most often, users dilute it with water and apply it with a cotton swab on their stains, as it seems to work very well. Apple cider vinegar is considered a good substitute for antibiotics, as it helps to treat bacterial infections.

You can probably use apple cider vinegar in two ways, one as an internal tonic and as a topical antibacterial solution.

Follow these steps and you can see significant results. First, take three tablespoons of apple cider vinegar in a bottle of water and mix them thoroughly. Then put a cotton swab on your face as an astringent.

Try using three different cotton balls on your face. Use one on the forehead, one on the cheeks and nose, and one on the chin. If you have a particularly oily nose, use one for this. This is to prevent the spread of bacteria from one site to your entire face, which would eventually cause more losses to other areas of your face. Although it is unusual, it is better to be confident than sorry.

Leave for about ten to fifteen minutes and rinse thoroughly with warm water. Then use a soft, clean towel to touch dry skin. Repeat this procedure three times a day to achieve maximum effect. For those who have severe forms of acne infection, you can apply a lower dose of the ACV diluted with three or four parts of water and leave for the night to do its job and wash the next day with warm water.

Keep in mind that if you want to apply apple cider vinegar, use a lower strength and leave it on the skin longer.

Another thing you can do is drink it with water with several spoons as a tonic every morning. This helps prevent acne rashes, reduce infection and dry inflammation. All you need to understand is that it does not have to taste pleasant to everyone. Try to drink like water and everything will be fine.

If you have really annoying prominent buttons, I advise you to mix one part of the LCA with three parts of water and dab on the button. Leave there for about fifteen minutes and rinse with warm water.

Some tips and warnings

- Never try to use apple cider vinegar at full power on the face as cases of skin lesions, irritations and burns have been reported. So pay attention to the use of this remedy, especially for those who have sensitive skin.
- Always use raw, unfiltered, unpasteurized apple cider vinegar. This will give you the best results.
- After using apple cider vinegar, dab a little tea tree oil on the acne. Tea tree oil works miracles for skin healing.
- If you are allergic to apples, apple cider vinegar is not for you.
- Do not use in combination with other acne medications. This will lead to complications and excessive drying of the skin.
- When using apple cider vinegar, it is better to start with the weakest combination of four parts of water. If it suits you, work on thicker mixtures. This means reducing the amount of water.
- Tingling is quite normal when using apple cider vinegar, but if you start to feel burning sensations, rinses it immediately with cool water.

Rounded and my conclusion

Everything about apple cider vinegar was very positive, except for the bitterness of vinegar, which you need to take carefully when applying to the face. I would recommend starting with a lower dose and then moderate it to a higher strength as you adapt to the current solution.

It is normal to feel tingling as it suggests it works. However, if you begin to feel the effects of burning, immediately wash off and reduce the strength of the stroke. For best results, use a water-based moisturizer for application to the skin after each stroke treatment. This is to prevent the skin from becoming too dehydrated due to the astringent properties of LCA.

I would like to point out that although apple cider vinegar can remove some superficial bacteria on the skin, it is not a long-term solution that can really stick acne to the root. There are almost many causes of acne, and bacteria are one of them.

It is more or less suitable for those who have mild to moderate acne and can see results in a few weeks. In severe cases, healing can take a long time. Have patience and you will reign over the world! The good thing is that you do it naturally and certainly don't burn your pockets while you do it.

All this makes sense to try this inexpensive home remedy before switching to more expensive products. Even if you have to, the severity of your acne condition would improve and you should not spend much time undergoing medical procedures provided by a dermatologist.

Can Apple Cider Vinegar Cure Toenail Fungus?

Apple cider vinegar is very popular among a large circle of people who are confident in natural home treatments. They want to choose, because apple cider vinegar from cider turned out to be one of the most effective natural drugs for the treatment of nail fungus. However, there are people who do not support the treatment of nail fungus compared to other treatment options. Here are two contra views. Go!

Apple cider vinegar can cure nails:

People with a slight degree of nail infection have shown that apple cider vinegar works well. Another advantage for their affirmation is their choice at the initial level of nail infection. Another thing is the easy availability of vinegar, which pleases them with what they have achieved to cure the infection. They found that this could prevent the spread of infection on the nails or nails. Another thing in support of the statement is a low price compared to other home treatment samples.

Apple cider vinegar cannot cure the infection of the nails on the legs:

Here the authenticity of apple cider vinegar is discussed differently. People who used vinegar without hope to heal the fungal infection are promoted to Tom-tom's propaganda, that a person may have a chance to heal the infected nail. Experts argue that this home remedy is not effective in the treatment of fungal nails as expected with Rapid Action. It says that vinegar cannot kill bacteria of all kinds. Vinegar restrictively states that it cannot guarantee the complete elimination of fungal spread. Vinegar must be mixed with hydrogen peroxide, which means that vinegar cannot fight the nail fungus on its own. Antagonists take their faith in the negative end the rumor that apple cider vinegar is best for severe cases of acne and is not suitable for the removal of nail fungus.

What is your choice?

Now you can analyze whether the treatment at home with vinegar suits you or not. It's up to you to decide on the safety of vinegar or with someone else to cure a nail infection.

Whatever your attitude to the work of apple cider vinegar, you need to know some measures when choosing this option.:

- Use diluted vinegar for mild infections and undiluted form for severe attacks
- Undiluted vinegar can cause skin irritation and sometimes burns.
- The application should last only a few minutes, say 10 minutes.
- Wash later with cold water and keep dry with a soft cloth.

- Apply vinegar exactly to the area of the infected nail, without spreading to close the skin.

Apple Cider Vinegar in Treatment of Cellulite

Cellulite is fat deposited under the surface of the skin around the hips, buttocks and thighs. Women of all races are affected by cellulite. It is observed mainly in obese women, but does not contain exclusively lean women. Although cellulite at least does not indicate a disease, it is often worrying for aesthetic reasons.

The skin contains strips of elastic tissue that go from the skin to the deeper layers of muscle tissue. These bands are inelastic and as fat deposited in the subcutaneous area the only way to move is to swell on the surface of the skin. The connective tissue tries to keep the skin in place, giving Dimple effect to the skin. The formation of cellulite is mainly due to an imbalance in the metabolism of fatty acids. Other factors, such as lack of physical activity and poor nutrition, are also responsible for the deposition of cellulite. Another factor contributing to the formation of cellulite is poor blood and lymph circulation, which leads to the accumulation of toxins in the body.

Many remedies are available for cellulite therapy and natural remedies are favored because of their safety profile. Apple cider vinegar is one of the natural remedies used to treat cellulite, which has been known for more than two thousand years in weight loss therapies.

Natural apple cider vinegar (ACV) is produced by crushing fresh, organic apples and allowing them to ripen in wooden barrels. This increases the natural fermentation and the vinegar ripens. Is a bacterial agent that is natural and effective that contains many essential minerals and trace elements such as potassium, calcium, magnesium, phosphorus, chlorine, sodium, sulfur, copper, iron, silicon and fluorine that are essential for a healthy body.

The role of apple cider vinegar in cellulite therapy

- or apple cider vinegar strengthens the immune system and heals many infections. It also increases the metabolic rate of the body and promotes thermogenesis.
- or as a result of an increase in basal metabolism leads to an increase in fat burning, which, as a result, balances cholesterol and causes weight loss.
- or other micronutrients present in apple cider vinegar such as vitamin B6 and lecithin also contribute to weight loss. While, weight loss is an essential aspect of apple cider vinegar cellulite therapy becomes extremely useful.
- or apple cider vinegar also helps to get rid of excess fluid accumulated in the body by helping to improve blood circulation.
- or it is also known to limit appetite.
- or apple cider vinegar is available in the form of capsules or liquids. Capsules can be taken only twice a day, and if necessary, they can be increased to three doses per day. The liquid form can be used as two tablespoons in a glass of water, taken before each meal.

Benefits of apple cider vinegar is that it is a natural remedy with proven effectiveness since ancient times in reducing weight apart from the fact that it is easy to use and effective.

Can Apple Cider Vinegar Help Fade Age Spots?

There are literally hundreds of products that should help mitigate the age spots sold on the market these days. Perhaps the abundance of products available today is the reason why those who suffer from age spots find it difficult to find the ideal treatment.

If you are one of those who cannot find proper treatment in faded age spots, you can consider using apple cider vinegar. It is a natural treatment that can help relieve the stitches.

This vinegar is made from fresh apples. They are crushed until the juice is extracted. Crushed apples ripen in a wooden barrel. This makes apple juice more refined than ordinary distilled vinegar sold on the market.

It contains many minerals, including calcium, copper, fluorine, chlorine, magnesium, potassium and sodium. These minerals are necessary for our health.

How Can Age Spots Fade?

It is not only a remedy for pigmentation spots, it can also help fight the effects of skin aging. It contains sulfur, which improves the health of your skin. It prevents the loss of the essential components of the dermis, which repair skin damage caused by the sun. Prolonged use of this treatment can relieve pigmentation spots.

Throw a medium-sized onion into your food processor. Mix to a delicate consistency. Put the onion on the cheese cloth and squeeze the juice. Mix one part of the onion juice and one part of apple cider vinegar. Apply this mixture directly to the points. Massage for about 30 seconds, then the solution can really penetrate the skin. Leave it there for about 30 minutes before washing with warm water.

You can accelerate the healing of the skin by combining this treatment with a natural moisturizer. Look for a moisturizer that contains natural ingredients such as Extrapone Nutgrass, Phytessence Wakame and Maracuja.

Extrapone Nutgrass is a component that contains effective lighting properties. This ingredient focuses on darker areas of the body and brightens them until they match the color of the skin complexion. It also works to improve the structure of the dermis.

Phytessence Wakame is a kind of Japanese algae that can reduce harmful enzymes. Get rid of these enzymes, as they attack hyaluronic acid, an acid that provides moisture to collagen proteins.

Apple Cider Vinegar for Weight Loss

Is A Diet Of Apple Cider Vinegar Good For Weight Loss?

Yes, the apple cider vinegar diet is certainly good for weight loss. Why is that? Because it is a natural drink for weight loss, and you can easily prepare it at home. This is a home remedy and was the grandmother's favorite remedy for a number of diseases. In addition, it is good for weight loss, apple cider vinegar is good for digestion, hypertension, hypercholesterolemia and many other conditions.

Is apple cider vinegar the best and how does it work?

The best is raw and organic. Why is that? Because it is in a natural state and its goodness is preserved. You can get it in pasteurized form. However, in this form, much of the basic resource and natural goodness is destroyed. In addition, it has been proven over the centuries that natural cider provides more effective weight loss results.

Those who use apple cider vinegar are of the opinion that it improves metabolism. They believe that it helps the body function better and this results in better burning of calories. There are others who have found that it burns fat and keeps appetite under control.

How to prepare a drink? It is better to mix it with warm water. Take a glass of wine or a favorite drink. How much do you drink? The recommended amount is two teaspoons per glass of water. For taste and many believe, for the best results, add two teaspoons of natural honey. How many glasses of this mixture should you consume? From seven to eight glasses of water considered a daily need, drink at least three with a mixture of apple cider vinegar.

Be very careful if you have a condition that can be aggravated by the content of sour apple cider vinegar.

The mixture is diluted if necessary. Don't take it well. If you are taking medications, it is better to consult your doctor.

Is the cider diet enough? Nope. This could just be part of your diet. Your weight loss program as a whole should consist of diet and exercise. Your diet should consist of eating the right kind. Exercises should be especially good for burning fat. Looking at the overall weight loss solution, look for the one that has the right combination of diet and exercise

Raw Apple Cider Vinegar Good for Weight Loss

For years, the vigorous exercise techniques, endless diets, diet pills and even extreme diets are the first things that come to mind when we all want to lose weight. But today you will learn that probably the best and most effective loss this unwanted fat can only be in your kitchen cupboard. It may sound too good to be true, but the fact is that raw apple cider vinegar was the reason for a number of successful weight loss stories for many years.

The funny thing is that no one knows why raw apple cider vinegar benefits weight loss and that includes years of scientific research and tests that have already been made to try to help find a suitable reason. Basically, the desire for consumption is mainly due to the success and a satisfied experience of others who have already tried and tested their abilities.

That is, there are theories that people have based on raw apple cider vinegar and how it actually helps with weight loss. Some have mentioned the possibility that they believe that you burn excess calories in the body, which helps the body get rid of these unwanted weights. Others believe that the metabolic rate increases dramatically and causes energy to produce even faster food in the body.

Another option could be that, as the reports mention, raw apple cider vinegar cleanses the liver, which seems to be a very important part of the human body, when it comes to helping with weight loss.

A recent study showed that consumption of raw apple cider vinegar before meals or even during meals would help individuals feel more sated, and thus prevent overeating. Even when he said it, it was only a small study and much more tests and experiments must be conducted on people, with the aim to find a definitive answer on the extent to which the raw apple cider vinegar really helps with weight loss.

Raw apple cider vinegar can be consumed in various ways, for example by adding a part into a glass of juice or even pure water. Other means can be consumed in a tablet or in the form of a capsule. Keep in mind that when you consume tablets or capsules, you can also consume other external vitamins, such as lecithin, which is a kind of vitamin B6 and works with a more pronounced effect on your body.

In addition to helping with weight loss raw apple cider vinegar has many other benefits and comes with many rich vitamins and minerals. One of the other main benefits, that heals, if not at least improve many health problems, such as lowering blood pressure due to the vinegar containing potassium. It also contains essential fiber and useful for the absorption of cholesterol, which can cause heart problems. Pain in the neck, arthritis pain and even diabetes are just some of the diseases that can be improved and even cured by eating a raw apple cider vinegar.

Like everything in this world, there are always two sides to the story. Which is the good side and the bad side. Unfortunately, raw apple cider vinegar and in this case it mentioned on his good side, also has its negative side. The risk that arises from the consumption of raw apple cider vinegar, is damage to the teeth, mouth or even throat of an individual due to the high content of acids. So, always be sure to dilute raw apple cider vinegar in juice or water before consumption. Take the necessary measures in terms of everything you do, and in this case it does not differ. Be sure to contact your local doctor or nutritionist if you suffer from serious health conditions before going on the consumption of raw apple cider vinegar for weight loss.

Apple Cider Vinegar Weight Loss and Benefits

You tried a lot of diets and you were frustrated with your results. Wouldn't it be nice to find something you can do every day to make it easier for you to lose weight or keep your weight? What if something was cheap, simple and excellent even for your overall health? Adding apple cider vinegar to weight loss can be the right thing to do. You can use it to lose weight and improve your overall health.

The use of apple cider vinegar for health and weight loss has a long history. The ancient Egyptians used it for centuries. Hippocrates, the father of Medicine used it almost exclusively for the treatment of all kinds of diseases. Many people and modern specialists who are aware of Health use it and recommend using it too.

The best type is raw, unfiltered, and made from organic apples. There are many nutrients and compounds in this type that are beneficial. It contains tons of vitamins and minerals that support the immune system, promote healthy brain function, and increase metabolism. It also promotes good oral health, helps wound healing, increases energy levels, and can reduce muscle and joint pain.

Several studies have been conducted which suggest that, with anywhere from one to three teaspoons of apple cider vinegar with water before each meal can reduce blood sugar after a meal. This reduces the amount of insulin needed in the body to treat ingested carbohydrates or sugars. It is useful for diabetics, and makes it less likely that the body stores excess calories in the form of fat. This makes fat loss and weight loss much easier.

While apple cider vinegar is acidic, it has alkalizing effect on the body when taken orally. The modern diet, which is full of processed foods, tends to leave the body more acidic. This imbalance of pH can cause many health problems. Too acidic environment makes your body more susceptible to infections caused by bacteria and fungi. It has been proved that apple cider vinegar also has antibiotics, antifungal agents, and antiseptic properties. In addition, it can help reduce hypercholesterolemia, and reduce water retention, thereby helping to reduce high blood pressure.

It also has other benefits for weight loss such as curb appetite and help with proper excretion. Therefore, when you use the apple cider vinegar weight loss, it also helps the body achieve proper pH balance, fight off infections and improve overall health. Weight loss of apple cider vinegar can only be a thing that keeps away from the doctor. Try it yourself and see how it can benefit you.

The Natural Solution: Apple Cider Vinegar Benefits for Beauty

Apple cider vinegar, sometimes called apple cider vinegar or ACV, is made from apple cider or cider. It has become very popular due to its many health benefits and beauty properties. Since the potassium content is high, it is better to consult a health professional before taking apple cider vinegar. Even if you can make your own apple cider vinegar, you will find it in its natural state, in any store, with healthy food. Let's explore some of the benefits of apple cider vinegar.

How to use apple cider vinegar

Apple cider vinegar can promote healthier skin and hair, as well as beneficial to health. For more specific ways by which apple cider can help treat specific ailments, contact a nutritionist who will be better prepared to answer specific questions. For more general use, you can try apple cider vinegar in some of the following ways.

Internal use

Research has shown that stroke can help the body in its daily functions, as well as fight colds and flu. It helps digestion, lowers bad cholesterol, strengthens the heart, lowers blood pressure and stabilizes blood sugar. It also contains antioxidants that help fight certain types of cancer. He can heal the stomach by daily drinking tonic.

To make your daily tonic, mix equal parts of apple cider vinegar and honey in a glass of water. Usually a tablespoon of apple cider vinegar and a tablespoon of honey in 8 oz of hot or cold water would be a general, but do not be afraid to change this recipe, based on personal preferences. There are other ways to drink it. You can add it to apple juice or add a little fresh cinnamon to neutralize its taste (some coffees serve the Apple with cinnamon).

External use

If your feet hurt, take a bath. Put half a cup of apple cider vinegar in a bath of warm water. Move your fingers and let your feet soak for a few minutes. Foot bath is a great way to relax before going to bed.

If your body is too acidic, take an acetic bath. To restore the acid-base balance of your body, add 1 to 2 cups of apple cider vinegar in a warm bath. Soak the body for about 45 minutes. In addition to cleansing the body of excess acid, a vinegar bath helps anyone with dry or irritated skin, feel soft.

If the baths are not for you, consider mixing a cup of each ACV and hot water in a spray bottle. After the shower, spray the entire body with a mixture. Wait a few minutes and rinse. Your whole body will feel refreshed.

Other benefits of apple cider vinegar include its local use on different parts of the body, especially on the face. For deep cleansing of the steamed face, add 3 tablespoons of apple cider vinegar in a saucepan of boiling water and tilt the face over it. Cover your head with a towel for a few minutes so that the Steam opens the pores and releases dirt from the surface of the skin.

Commercial products on the market

In addition to the natural form of apple cider vinegar, there are many commercial products. These products include body washing and preparations for hair and face. Taking apple cider vinegar in the natural state is just as beneficial, if not better, than these products.

Warning

Since apple cider vinegar is very acidic, never drink directly. Always dilute with water. After drinking apple cider vinegar, rinse your mouth with water. Also, do not brush your teeth right away, as it could grind your vinegar into enamel. A great way to prevent apple cider vinegar from touching your teeth is to drink it with a straw. ACV tablets are an excellent alternative to liquid, although they do not work so quickly. Also, avoid eye contact with apple cider vinegar as the acid will burn and blush your eyes

The benefits of apple cider vinegar seem endless. These simple methods and ways to use LCA are all large and inexpensive. Most importantly, they have proven methods beneficial to your body and the environment. As long as you use it carefully and for recognized and healthy purposes, the benefits of apple cider vinegar will continue to reveal themselves. Try it yourself.

Apple Cider Vinegar Cures: The Power of Acid

If you've ever heard of apple cider vinegar cures, but were wondering if it was just female stories, don't ask yourself anymore. Apple cider vinegar and its use are real and have been tested over the centuries. It's time to start taking this powerful drug.

The acid in vinegar has been used successfully over and over again to help many skin conditions, including bacterial proliferation, to remove the heavy residue left by soaps and shampoos, and even help with things like reducing acne breaks. It improves hair and skin by helping to maintain a younger appearance and is a useful disinfectant.

So, if you want younger skin, less acne, shiny and beautiful hair, you need to start using apple cider vinegar. If you do not suffer from Candida, vaginal yeast infection, or a sports itch, then you need this natural remedy.

By placing apple cider vinegar and a little salt in the bath water, you will make the water neutral, making it a more natural bath that is perfect for feeling the skin and body. It is useful to take apple cider vinegar during a trip abroad, when there are possible problems with contaminated food and water. The introduction of vinegar into water kills many types of bacteria and was used in ancient times for this purpose. Similarly, drinking a few full teaspoons of apple cider vinegar in 8 ounces of water just before a meal can help kill food-related bacteria by helping to reduce the possibility of food poisoning.

Here's more cider.

Bleeding: for hundreds of years, doctors have vinegar to treat wounds and stop excessive bleeding. With cuts and nosebleeds, it is necessary to soak a cotton swab in vinegar and put it on a cup or place it in a bleeding nose. Many are also advised to take internally before and after surgery.

Allergies: it is considered that apple cider vinegar, if taken as a daily tonic, can improve immune function and improve metabolism, which will help reduce many types of allergic reactions. While, asthma and arthritis are perceived by some as an allergic reaction, it is often recommended for these conditions.

Bone health: apple cider vinegar contains magnesium and Manganese Minerals that improve health. It also contains traces of mineral boron, which helps the body metabolize calcium and magnesium, which helps the bones to strengthen.

Blood pressure: apple cider vinegar is a good source of potassium, which balances sodium in the body by helping to reduce blood pressure.

Always consult your doctor before taking these or all natural remedies.

Apple Cider Vinegar for Candida

Looking for information about apple cider vinegar for Candida? In this book you will find information about apple cider vinegar and yeast infection, as well as whether apple cider vinegar kills Candida.

For many people who are concerned about constant yeast infections, there is a good chance that you have stumbled upon the remedies that suggest using this to kill yeast infections. You may wonder why something that is usually used as a cooking ingredient is used to clean the infection, but the truth is that apple cider vinegar is one of the remedies most powerful for yeast infection out there. It does not matter whether the yeast infection is vaginal or occurs under the arms or in the form of fat. There are several reasons why you can use vinegar and apple cider, and you will find that for many people this is the best solution that is available to them.

One of the reasons why it is so effective is its alkaline nature. Not only does a small amount of it bring your body's pH levels online, it can also kill the Candida fungus that causes yeast infection. It works to protect your body, as well as reduce the toxicity of different compounds by converting the toxin into something that is less toxic. This in turn can strengthen the immune system and prevent getting yeast infections in the future.

When you try to determine whether it kills Candida or not, you will find that there are many important minerals in vinegar, as well as trace elements such as potassium, magnesium, chlorine, copper and iron, which you could get daily. It can help your body collect and fight infections, as well as vitamin C and vitamin A, which is also in it.

Looking at the use of apple cider vinegar and yeast infection, the most common way to do this is to apply it on a clean, dry cloth and hold it against the affected area for about twenty minutes. Then you can rinse it, make sure that your body is well dried. You can also add a cup of apple cider vinegar to a shallow bath for twenty minutes of soaking, or two cups for a more complete bath. Do not forget to change the treatment as you think best and that if in a few weeks you do not react to apple cider vinegar, you may try something else.

Take the time to see if apple cider vinegar kills Candida and why so many people rave about apple cider vinegar for Candida; you may find that you have a drug you were looking for!

Apple Cider Vinegar for BV Treatment Method and Uses

Apple cider vinegar has many uses. Some people use it in cooking, some use it in cleaning and some of it is also used as a medicine or home remedy. For Example, some people use apple cider vinegar for BV relief.

BV, or bacterial vaginosis, is not a funny condition. This can cause both internal and external vagina to become swollen, painful and itchy. It can also cause discharge and unpleasant odors from the vagina. During this time you may experience cramps, swelling or even bleeding associated with your BV. This can really make you sad and definitely kill your sex life. So this is a condition where most women rush to heal.

Kill Bacteria:

A traditional medical way to cure BV, which is a bacterial infection, is to kill the attacking bacteria. Your doctor may advise you to do so by taking antibiotics. However, antibiotics kill all bacteria and the thing that many women do not understand is that a woman's vagina must contain healthy bacteria that protect it.

Change Balance:

The reason apple cider vinegar works just like BV treatment is that it is slightly acidic. Therefore, it has the power to change the pH balance of the vagina just so that good bacteria stay healthy and prevent bad bacteria from developing. Therefore, you can slightly adjust the vaginal environment, rather than erase all bacteria with antibiotics.

Spa Vinegar:

If you are going to use cider vinegar to alleviate the symptoms of BV, an easy way to do this is to take a bath of cider vinegar. Start with a warm, shallow bath. Then mix about half a cup of vinegar with water from the bath. Be careful not to add too much vinegar because it might cause a strong burning sensation, when sitting in the bath.

A bath of apple cider vinegar can be useful, but you should not do it too often. Remember, you just want to restore balance in your vagina. Turning the stairs too far in the opposite direction could only exacerbate your problems.

Vinegar Shower:

As an acetic bath, the acetic shower should be sufficiently diluted. A teaspoon of apple cider vinegar in two cups of water should fit. Also, as with vinegar bath, you should not take a shower too often. Once a day is enough for work.

Drink Vinegar:

Drinking apple cider vinegar is a good way to prevent BV, although it may not be useful as a bath or a shower, as regards the management of existing epidemic BV. Use apple cider vinegar for BV relief, especially if you want to drink, however, it should be done carefully. Since it is slightly acidic, you do not need or need a large amount of preparation in the body. So use it in moderation and you should find that it can bring much needed BV relief.

Apple Cider Vinegar for Bacterial Vaginosis - Treatment Methods

Methods of treating bacterial vaginosis must appear for hundreds of years. After all, this is a natural substance. So, it was here long before modern medicines were invented.

Many Uses:

One of the reasons cider vinegar lasts so long is that it has many uses. For example, it has antibacterial and slightly acidic properties. Thus, it is a good natural remedy for many diseases, including BV. Thanks to these properties, vinegar is an excellent cleaner. Not only that, but also it can be an ingredient in many cooking recipes.

A natural way to treat BV:

Another reason why apple cider vinegar has remained so popular is that it is a natural way to treat BV. It is slightly acidic, which can help restore the pH level in your body. However, it is not acidic enough to be harmful. In addition, antibiotic therapy tends to reduce BV symptoms only for a short time, not permanently. In fact, in general, natural remedies and herbal remedies are much more suitable for supporting your body than chemicals made by man.

Three Ways to Use Apple Cider Vinegar:

There are many ways to treat or prevent bacterial vaginosis using apple cider vinegar. The best way to prevent BV is to drink every day just a little diluted with water. However, you should not drink more than one teaspoon in a large glass of water twice a day. In fact, once a day is probably enough.

Of course, you can choose and rinse with this vinegar, which is a good way to help cure an existing case of BV. Two cups of water and a teaspoon of apple cider vinegar should be enough. You should only joke once a day. Excessive rinsing can lead to the loss of good vaginal bacteria, as well as bad. Therefore, it is important not to have anything more than is necessary.

The third option is that you can simply take a bath in apple cider vinegar, but not in a full bath. Use about half to one stirred in a shallow bath. If you use too much vinegar, you will feel a strong burning sensation in your vaginal area. In addition, you risk killing all the good bacteria in the vagina, which is never a good idea.

Use More Than Just Apple Cider Vinegar:

If you want some great tips for preventing or treating BV, you should try immediate relief of bacterial vaginosis. This is a comprehensive program that offers a unique insight into the treatment of BV by all natural methods. Considering all things, the system can help you support your body and get rid of bacterial vaginosis forever. After all, if you want complete relief from BV, it is necessary to use more than these methods of treatment with vinegar bacterial vaginosis.

Looking For Apple Cider Vinegar Dandruff Cure?

An old folk remedy, apple cider vinegar has been used for centuries as a remedy for dandruff. I'll show you a quick way to get home.

Dandruff is caused by yeasts like Malassezia Globosa or Pityrosporum Ovale that like the oil secretion from the glands around the hair follicles. These yeast fungi feed on oil (sebum) secreted by the glands and clog the pores of the head. Some people are sensitive to yeast and it irritates their skin, trying to get rid of the fungus flakes, leading to dandruff.

Apple cider vinegar will kill the fungus and help restore the correct acid / alkaline balance of the head. It will also add a great shine to your hair.

To properly Apple cider vinegar to the dandruff remedy, try the following recipe below:

Wash your hair with a mild shampoo at a balanced pH. it is not necessary to use dandruff shampoo, since apple cider vinegar will gradually get rid of the problem of dandruff.

Mix two parts of apple cider vinegar and one part of warm water. Adding a few drops of essential oils, such as lavender or rosemary will help clean the scalp and add fragrance to the hair. (Do not forget to glue test oils for allergies and always consult your doctor if you are pregnant).

Pour the mixture directly with clean hair or put it in a vial and spray on the head. Massage and allow the mixture to dry on the hair. It is not necessary to rinse it (if the smell does not bother you).

For more stubborn dandruff, try a stronger mixture, such as the ratio of vinegar and water. You can also try to use undiluted vinegar and apply directly to the scalp. We let it act for about 15 minutes, then we wash the cider with a mild shampoo at a balanced pH.

You will get the best results when using raw, unfiltered apple cider vinegar to treat dandruff. Lemon juice can also be used instead of apple cider vinegar.

In these means there is an acid that helps to return the skin to chemical balance.

The remedy for dandruff cider is an excellent home remedy for getting rid of dandruff, and on the skin it is easier than many shampoos from the shelves.

There are many remedies for itchy scalp and dandruff that you can do from the comfort of your own home.

Apple Cider Vinegar GERD

Is there really such a thing as GERD apple cider vinegar? Lucky for! Many people suggest that this type of vinegar is the newest natural remedy for gastro esophageal reflux (acid reflux). But is it really working?

As a natural health expert, my research team and I have examined hundreds of drugs and found many charlatans. On the other hand, my research team also found drugs that outperform drugs and antacids.

At the end of this book you will learn why you want to get rid of antacids and try this new drug.

Why apple cider vinegar (ACV)?

Even if it tastes terrible, you may have heard a lot of positive things about apple cider vinegar. Many of you know at least one elderly person who drinks alcohol every day, claiming that he has not been sick for 20 years. You can even drink it every time you feel a cold. The truth is that this type of vinegar is full of vitamins, minerals and acid!

But does it really work for RGO (also known as acid reflux)?

Yeah! And let me explain why! Did you know that most acid reflux is caused by too little acid in the stomach? It makes sense when you think about how it works. If your stomach does not produce enough acid for digestion, then more food (and gas) will remain in the stomach for a longer period of time...without properly digesting.

So, apple cider vinegar is so acidic that it immediately begins to digest food in the stomach and very quickly relieves heartburn.

Apple cider vinegar RGO medicine

How is this type of medication used?

You don't need a lot of apple cider vinegar to make this remedy work! One or two chips can do this. It would be equal to about 1-2 teaspoons.

After drinking vinegar, you will notice a slight burning sensation for about 5 seconds, but then it should disappear and you will notice almost immediate relief. And the good thing is that this remedy will work for days. (Antacids can only act for a few hours.)

It is also recommended to buy the best quality vinegar possible. The Bragg brand has been a very popular choice of our customers. Cheaper brands have not been so successful.

Unfortunately, you will notice the terrible taste when you try this drug for the first time. Fortunately, the taste is not worth it. However, you can dilute the vinegar by adding a glass of water and add honey. This will make the mixture easier and easier to enjoy.

100% Guaranteed Remedy against Acid Reflux

Believe it or not, this is only 1 of nearly 40 + acid reflux remedies that have been studied and proven to help cure GERD naturally. If you want to cure RGO constantly using simple ingredients you can find in any grocery store.

Arthritis and Apple Cider Vinegar

The use of apple cider vinegar to improve a wide range of health problems is certainly not new.

You know, Oxymel has been a pillar of home remedies and simple healing for centuries.

Oxymel is simply a mixture of equal parts of apple cider vinegar with raw honey. It is used twice a day, dilute a tablespoon in a glass of water and take the first thing in the morning and the last thing before bedtime.

There are slight differences in the recipe because some people add crushed seeds of fennel and other species, as well as crushed garlic. Similarly, some people heat the mixture with syrup while others mix everything and let it rest a day before use.

As I know, Oxymel has been used in my family for many generations and has always been associated with arthritis as pain and other joint pain conditions.

But there are many reports that claim that apple cider vinegar is useful in other diseases, such as acne, dandruff, dyspepsia, for detoxing after a period of self neglect, dissolve calcium deposits that are painful in the body, hay fever, neutralize harmful bacteria, which can be found in food, digestive disorders, and the list can last forever.

If all this is true, I really do not know, but the only thing I can say is that arthritis and apple cider vinegar are a combination of earnings. Use apple cider vinegar to reduce arthritis pain and receive extra benefits as a bonus!

Symptoms of arthritis include pain and limited joint function. Inflammation of the joints with arthritis is characterized by joint stiffness, swelling, redness and heat. All these symptoms can be alleviated or eliminated by taking oxymel twice a day. At least that's what I think.

But like I said, I have to think about it. Perhaps faith is an important part of the healing ability of any medicine. I have seen many members of my Oxymel family with plain believe that this simple action will help their painful condition, and it certainly did. Some time ago, I recommended this home remedy to a friend who was extremely skeptical; and although twice a day to eat apple cider vinegar for a period of more than three weeks, did not notice an improvement with your arthritis pain.

This is not a cure for arthritis, and apple cider vinegar should not be stopped, or you will again feel the symptoms of arthritis. You need to take it every day to see continuous relief and always consult your doctor about the treatment of the disease.

In addition to drinking oxymel, soaking arthritis of the joints in warm apple cider vinegar (1 part of apple cider vinegar to 6 parts of warm water) can bring additional relief.

Apple cider vinegar is safe, if you do not have an allergy to yeast, in which case you can not in any way use this home remedy. in addition, some people have concerns about the side effects of vinegar on the sensitivity of teeth and erosion of enamel, so they recommend adding baking soda to make the preparation slightly alkaline. I do not add, because although I am very confident with apple cider vinegar, I have many doubts about the side effects of baking soda itself. What I do is I have a mouthwash gently after taking the oxymol. But you can avoid these problems by making the tablet supplement available on the market.

How to Use Apple Cider Vinegar for Yeast Infection

The use of apple cider vinegar for yeast infection is one of the most effective methods of treating this problem. Read how it works...

Yeast infection, also known as candidiasis, is caused by the spread of certain fungi called "candida albicans" that can affect many parts of the body, for example, the skin, mouth, intestines and vaginal area.

But apple cider vinegar is an effective remedy for candidiasis: it contains natural enzymes that help control the growth of Candida fungi. At the same time, it also promotes the friendly growth of bacteria that keep Candida fungi even tighter under control.

Apple cider vinegar for oral yeast infection

Sometimes infection can occur in the mouth and is commonly known as thrush.

This infection causes white and cream injuries and wounds on the inner cheeks or under / over the tongue.

Oral thrush can be extremely painful, causing bleeding and problems with food, chewing and swallowing.

A very effective way to combat thrush is to use apple cider vinegar as a mouthwash...

Dilute 2 teaspoons of raw, unfiltered water to a size of 8 ounces. Clean the water, rinse it in your mouth, then spit or swallow. Most people prefer to spit.

Repeat 2-3 times a day for about 3 days or until the symptoms disappear.

You can use apple cider vinegar for yeast infection on the skin

Yeast can also affect the skin, especially inside and around the inguinal area, between the toes and fingers, under the chest, under all other folds of the skin and under the nail beds.

These infections appear as rashes blisters that lose fluid or red, dry bumps, which itch.

Raw apple cider vinegar is recommended to relieve all the discomfort and pain of candidiasis of the skin...

You can use it as a bath: empty two cups filled with vinegar in a full warm bath completely soak the affected area.

Stay in the water for half an hour or two, then repeat this treatment every day until the symptoms disappear.

Apple cider vinegar is especially effective for yeast intestinal infections

In some cases, infection can occur in the intestinal tract where when the yeast begins to multiply and spread it can cause toxic side effects.

There are many causes of intestinal infections, but the most common are excessive use of antibiotics, stress, decreased immunity, hormonal imbalance and poor nutrition.

Symptoms of this infection include: joint and muscle pain, headache, depression, irritability, anxiety, rash, intestinal cramps, diarrhea, severe gas, bloating, heartburn, belching and oral thrush.

ACD can greatly help this problem by killing toxic yeast and balancing the friendly intestinal flora in the intestine...

Drink two tablespoons of apple cider vinegar diluted in 8 ounces. Water two or three times a day. Repeat every day until the symptoms disappear.

Apple cider vinegar and vaginal yeast infection

Incredibly, yeast vaginal infection affects at least 75% of women at some point in their lives. Even worse, about half of them will have recurrent infections.

Most women suffering from this particular infection experience burning, itching and redness of the outer part of the vagina, white or yellow discharge and some discomfort in their pelvic area.

Apple cider vinegar is used to treat this type of yeast infection in the same way as a yeast infection for the previously described skin, that is, soak in a warm bath containing two cups of apple cider vinegar.

You can also use apple cider vinegar diluted with cold hot water as a shower: apply the shower twice a day for best results.

You need to be careful when buying apple cider vinegar for yeast infection: choose raw, unfiltered and unpasteurized vinegar for this purpose. This will bring you better results, because it has a higher nutritional value.

A Vinegar Remedy for Male Yeast Infection

Cider for male yeast infection? Does it work? Yes, according to many. For centuries, people with various diseases have sworn their effectiveness. And this is the same with yeast infection. Apple cider vinegar is used by men and women around the world to get relief from their yeast infections. Apple cider vinegar is one of the most popular and effective natural remedies for yeast infection available.

First, let's look together at what causes yeast infection. It is a yeast-like fungus called Candida albicans. This, of course, exists in most of us, without causing problems. It is kept under the control of favorable or good bacteria of your body. However, under certain conditions it is not effective enough, and Candida "develops" in the symptoms of yeast infection.

Many men and women seem that normal drug-based treatment does not work; the symptoms disappear for a minute and then come back. It is believed that the reason they have recurrent yeast infections is that the drugs treat only the symptoms, not the root or root causes (causes). And Candida fungi can become resistant to drugs.

Therefore, many men and women turn to natural home remedies, apple cider vinegar is one of the most popular.

Apple cider vinegar has antiseptic properties (among others), which help to calm itching and relieve pain and discomfort, for example, from a yeast infection of the penis. That's how you use it...

(1) in a slightly warm bath, add 2 cups of apple cider vinegar and turn to mix well. The "low" bath means enough water to ensure that the legs and penis are no longer covered. It will be necessary to soak for about 20-30 minutes. Discharge the foreskin to make sure that the head is properly soaked.

(2) you can also Mix 2 tablespoons of apple cider vinegar with 2 liters of warm water and gently moisten the affected area with cotton wool soaked in water / vinegar and mix.

(3) drinking a dilution of apple cider vinegar is good to help balance the good bacteria in the intestinal tract, and thus helps to prevent the Candida fungus, stormed there and potentially spreading yeast infection to other parts of the body. Just Mix 2 teaspoons of vinegar in 8 oz. a glass of water. Drink three times a day.

Apple cider vinegar can help with infection of male yeast. But it's just a piece of the puzzle. For complete recovery without relapse it is necessary to take into account other aspects, such as lifestyle, diet, etc. without them you have to deal only with the symptoms of a yeast infection, and not with the basic problems. But now you have seen that traditional drug treatment can not get all this. And more and more men and women go completely naturally.

A Natural Treatment for Yeast Infections

And the natural treatment of yeast infections is what more and more patients are looking for today. Tired of recurrent yeast infections, turning this natural treatment like apple cider vinegar to your infection. The latter do not have negative aspects of drug treatment and are much cheaper.

First, let's see why thousands of people are moving away from the traditional treatment of yeast infections...

Traditional treatment usually involves the use of local creams, gels and the intention behind it, local areas with symptoms. It deals with local symptoms, but not the cause. And since they are addicted to drugs, at work, fungi Candida albicans (the cause of infection) can accumulate and resist them. The result can be a mentally destructive recurrent yeast infection.

While the fungus Candida albicans are the cause of infection, something must happen to the fungus to overcome the "friendly" bacteria in your body, whose task is to keep the fungus under control. These basic or starting problems are things like diabetes, lowers the immune system, excessive use of antibiotics, stress, poor nutrition, etc.

Now let's look at the popular natural treatment of yeast infection...

One of the most effective is raw apple cider vinegar. But it must be raw, unrefined, unpasteurized, without additives. You are more likely to take it to a healthy store than to a supermarket. Check the label and / or ask the Wizard.

Why is such a popular natural treatment of yeast infection? Raw apple cider vinegar has antifungal properties that help fight Candida albicans. It contains such things as amino acids, minerals, trace elements (e.g. potassium, iron, calcium, etc.), vitamins, enzymes, etc. so the use of apple cider vinegar also helps your overall health.

You can drink it by mixing 2 teaspoons of 8 ounces a glass of cold water, three times a day. You can also use as a natural cocktail by adding 2 tablespoons per 2 liters of warm water. Or you can use it in the bath "sitz" by adding two cups of vinegar to a low, warm bath. Just enough water to cover your hips. Soak for about 20 minutes.

But if he can relieve discomfort and symptoms, his apple cider vinegar is unlikely to lead a permanent healing, without even addressing the underlying problems.

How to Use Apple Cider Vinegar to Clear Your Thrush

Apple cider vinegar is a well-known home remedy for thrush. Many sick people who are tired trying to eliminate their Thrush through the usual topical creams and pessaries, etc., turned to such natural remedies as apple cider vinegar. Thrush (also called yeast infection) is an infection caused by the proliferation of a yeast-like fungus called Candida Albicans. Most women suffer from vaginal thrush. Here you will find out how to use apple cider vinegar for vaginal thrush.

Apple cider vinegar has been successfully used as a natural remedy for a number of ailments for thousands of years. Trace elements, minerals, enzymes, beneficial bacteria, etc., found in raw apple cider vinegar represents its healing properties. And thrush is no exception.

But you need to make sure that it is raw, not distilled and not pasteurized, without additives and preservatives. You can get it in some grocery stores or supermarkets, but the best solution is your local health food store. Here's how to use it...

As a drink, mix two teaspoons of apple cider vinegar in a glass of water. Drink three times a day. This will help control Candida Albicans fungi in the intestine.

As a Topical Drug, you can take a shower with it. Just add two tablespoons of vinegar to two liters of warm water and lightly moisten with a cotton swab. Do it twice a day. Stop when symptoms disappear. Vinegar helps to rebalance vaginal pH (acidity), thus helping to control the growth of Candida fungi.

Many women prefer to take a bath. For a warm and low bath, add two cups of apple cider vinegar and sit in the bath for about twenty minutes. Open the labia of the vagina so that the hot solution can better reach the infection. If you can repeat twice a day until the symptoms of Thrush disappear.

Apple cider vinegar is a very popular home remedy for thrush. But this is just one of the many home remedies for thrush in use today. What women have found is that some work better than others, and what might work for one person might not work for another.

And there are other contradictory factors to consider. For example, some of the things that can help Candida fungi develop too are things like overuse of antibiotics, poor diet, steroids, compromised immune system, weight problems, medications, diabetes, etc., you will have to take all of these things into account to find a permanent cure for thrush.

Apple Cider Vinegar: Remedies Galore!

If you are looking for information about apple cider vinegar, you have come to the right place. This type of vinegar is what you get when you let cider brew in alcohol, then let the alcohol brew in vinegar. The substance that remains in vinegar is acetic acid, which gives vinegar its aroma and taste.

Acetic acid found in cider vinegar has been expanded to help with weight loss. Helps prevent accumulation of body fat and certain liver fats so it may help you achieve your weight loss goals. Regular consumption of acetic acid can help you reduce waist and abdominal areas.

Another folk remedy for which this vinegar was used helps people with diabetes. Several studies have shown that consuming apple cider vinegar before going to bed will bring much more favorable blood sugar in the morning. It also helps to increase the amount of good cholesterol and reduce the amount of fat in the blood.

If you suffer from dandruff, you can use apple cider vinegar to cure your problem. Mixing vinegar with water and inserting the mixture into the hair, it helps restore the acid balance on the head. This method is usually used only once or twice a week for fifteen minutes at a time.

Acne can also be helped with the use of apple cider vinegar. This solution goes in the same direction as the remedy for dandruff. Vinegar is mixed with water and a drop on the affected areas of the skin. But keep an eye on it. Vinegar can burn the skin if the mixture has too much vinegar.

You should be careful if you decide to use vinegar in your home remedies. If you drink vinegar, you risk damaging the throat and teeth. If you have low potassium levels or have osteoporosis, consult your doctor before taking vinegar in your diet. With excessive use, you can also damage the stomach and liver.

If you are always looking for more information about the benefits or risks of using apple cider vinegar, you can learn more by doing a quick online search. There are many resources that will tell you which means use vinegar and what you should look for. Stay informed!

So if you decide that you want to taste the apple cider vinegar for your own home remedy, take the time to consult with your doctor whether it is safe for you to use.

Knowing the risks and benefits of using vinegar will only help you make the right decision for you.

Apple Cider Vinegar Wart Removal

Skin tags or warts are a very common maintenance among men and women of all ages, but they are difficult to cure. A very popular method of treating warts in the comfort of your own home is the method of removing the wart from apple cider vinegar. Before considering the solution of the problem, it is important first of all to understand what the causes of warts are.

In general, warts are the result of a very contagious and difficult to eliminate human papillomavirus. This is due to the many forms of the virus that exist, and usually the location of the wart is determined by the type and nature of the virus that causes it. The Virus easily contracts through the broken skin in the form of cuts, and when another carrier touches these areas (skin to skin), the virus passes through. Although it is unpleasant and, depending on the location, embarrassing, these types of warts can be easily treated. The problem with such remedies as removing warts with apple cider vinegar is that they usually do not treat the cause of the problem, so there is a high probability that they will come back again.

Although warts around the genital area are the most embarrassing places (and cause the most pain), the most common tend to be the legs or hands. This is because many people share soaps and washing items within the family and when a family member is infected, it is very easy to pass on the infection.

There are a number of home remedies to combat warts one of the most common techniques is the removal of warts apple cider vinegar. Although this treatment can help patients reduce the problem, there is no permanent cure. I have suffered with skin tags for many years, I can sympathize with everyone who suffers from warts. In my case, skin tags in the armpits caused real problems, especially during the summer months. Warts and skin tags are easily aggravated by constant movement and can become very painful to the extent that physical exercise is avoided.

The problem with most home remedies, including removing warts apple cider vinegar, is that it usually stops the condition of repeating. Fortunately for me, there is now a new drug on the market that has incredible success in terms of removing warts and skin signs.

The best part of this new remedy is that a trip to the doctor or even to the hospital (with the scar) is not necessary since the treatment is something that can be used at home without resorting to surgery to cut skin tags. If you have already looked at frozen skin labels, this is not the treatment you want to undergo lightly. Not only does this new technique of removing warts deprive your body of warts, but also all forms of skin tags and even these embarrassing genital warts. Even more effective is that this type of treatment should be applied only once to the affected area and in a few days it is removed forever. No more fear of heat, just a permanent and rapid removal of warts.

Benefits to Using Apple Cider Vinegar for Your Dog's Health

I'm sure you've heard of the use of apple cider vinegar for natural remedies in people, but have you heard of using it for your dog's health? Apple cider vinegar can help with digestion, gas, constipation, bladder stones and urinary tract infections. It is used to scare off insects such as mosquitoes, fleas and tics. It can alleviate the condition of the skin and even remove the smell of skunk.

Many herbalists recommend the use of vinegar. It is recommended to buy vinegar based on whole apples cold pressed and organically grown, to benefit from the enzymes present in nature.

In its natural form, apple cider vinegar is a natural antibiotic, antiseptic and deodorant. It helps to remove tartar from teeth, prevents caries and hair loss (including scabies), prevents and cures gum disease.

Have I listed enough benefits to use apple cider vinegar?

The use of apple cider vinegar has many other advantages. It is known to reduce common infections, help the puppy, improve endurance, prevent muscle fatigue after exercise, increase resistance to diseases and protect against food poisoning. Apple cider vinegar is rich in vitamins, minerals and trace elements found in apples, especially potassium; it normalizes acid levels in the stomach, improves digestion and absorption of nutrients, reduces intestinal gases and fecal odors, helps cure constipation, relieves some of the symptoms of arthritis, and helps prevent bladder stones and urinary tract infections.

You can feed apple cider vinegar every day for your dog to be healthy. Add to food or water. You may need to gradually increase the dose. Start with a few drops and slowly increase each day until you reach the recommended daily dose below.

Recommended approximate quantities :

1 teaspoon-dogs up to 14 pounds

2 teaspoons-medium dogs-from 15 to 34 pounds

1 tablespoon-large dogs - £ 35 to £ 84

By mixing your dog's food or water, apple cider vinegar restores the acid / alkaline balance of its digestive tract, eliminating brown spots in the lawn. A good pH balance also helps to ward off fleas, black flies, ticks and other external pests. Your dog will be less likely to have ringworm, Staphylococcus, Streptococcus and scabies infections. If your dog already has these problems sponge your dog's skin with a mixture of equal parts of apple cider vinegar with the same amount of warm water. If you prefer, you can use this mixture in a spray bottle to completely immerse your dog.

Caution: do not use apple cider vinegar if the dog is sensitive or allergic to yeast or has a chronic yeast infection. Also, do not give dogs with irritated intestines.

How Soaking Gout Feet in Apple Cider Vinegar Can Relieve Gout

Gout is a form of arthritis and is probably the most painful form of arthritis it is. And as you probably know, GOUT occurs mostly in the feet particularly in the big joint at the base of the finger, which becomes swollen, inflamed and extremely painful.

Because of this, it completely disrupts your daily life, because it prevents you from walking as usual. That is why many people suffering from gout go to their doctor for the first sign of gout for treatment to relieve pain.

The medical profession largely offers medication-based treatments to reduce inflammation and relieve pain. They can also offer drugs that lower the level of uric acid in the blood to try to prevent further attacks.

Unfortunately, these drugs can have quite unpleasant side effects, and, they are effective only when taken. They can't work if you get out. Therefore, drugs to reduce uric acid are a long-term prospect.

Thus, people suffering from gout are increasingly taking advantage of many benefits of natural drugs for gout, many of which are. But there are too many. But many sick people use apple cider vinegar...

Dip drop feet in apple cider vinegar

Apple cider vinegar has been used since ancient times for a number of diseases and conditions, including gout treatment. But, of course, today with refined vinegar, etc., you need to pay attention to what apple cider vinegar you use.

It must be raw, undistilled, unpasteurized apple cider vinegar, the kind that most likely you will get from a medical warehouse or other specialized health care. Ask your assistant for an explanation. But you can recognize raw apple cider vinegar, because it will have a good amount of sediment - called "mother" - at the bottom of the bottle.

Soak the bottom of the feet to help relieve pain and reduce swelling, just add 1/2 cup of the raw cider to 3 cups of warm water in the pan. Plus, double or triple the ratio I just gave you. Immerse the hollow foot / foot for 25-30 minutes and, if necessary, repeat, warm up the water again.

Now, for more information, you can actually drink raw apple cider vinegar to change the pH of the blood, which can help reduce uric acid in the blood. For a Drink, Mix 3 teaspoons of vinegar in a large glass of water and drink 2-3 times a day. You can add a little honey to remove the "edge" of the taste if you want.

Try this completely natural remedy to bathe the bottom of the foot and see how it climbs. Don't forget to drink too much!

That said, because there are a lot of underlying triggers for gout and everyone is different, you need to get acquainted with all the natural gout remedies out there because apple cider vinegar is not the cure gout itself.

This is important, because if you can permanently stop recurring gout attacks from time to time, you run the risk of permanent joint damage, kidney damage, or even high blood pressure in the future.

3 Frequently Asked Questions You Should Know

Does the use of apple cider vinegar really work to cure acid reflux? Wondering if this is just another mythical remedy or the solution you are looking for? If so, then you want to read this article. This article will tell you why and how it can be a real savior for those who suffer from heartburn. After reading this, you will be convinced that you will use it to relieve reflux disease.

What does apple cider vinegar contain? How does it help me relieve the pain of heartburn?

Apple is the main ingredient, it is one of the most nutritious fruits that contain many vitamins and minerals such as pectin, beta-carotene, calcium, iron, phosphorus and potassium, as well as enzymes and amino acids.

Wait, amino acids? Wouldn't it add even more acid to the esophagus, which would further increase the burning sensation?

Contrary to popular belief, acid reflux occurs because there is not enough gastric acid to digest food. Lack of acid in the stomach causes relaxation of the lower sphincter of the esophagus (SLE) so that they release digested and acidic foods into the esophagus. Consuming apple cider vinegar, the acid level of the stomach becomes normal, and you will be able to properly digest food.

Here sucks! It tastes terrible! How can I drink?

Well, honestly, not only apple cider vinegar, the most effective natural remedies do not taste good if they are ingested directly. The correct dosage for regular consumption would be 1 teaspoon of vinegar with 8 ounces of water. 1 teaspoon of honey is recommended to neutralize the acidic aftertaste. In addition to direct consumption, you can also mix it with food (dressing, mayonnaise or sprinkled with chips and chips) or your regular tea.

As you can see in the 3 Most Frequently Asked Questions above, using apple cider vinegar to cure acid reflux is not a placebo effect. It really helps your metabolism. This simple home remedy may be able to help relieve the symptoms of gastric juice and heartburn. If this or any other medication is not effective in reducing symptoms, you should consult a doctor who specializes in the treatment of acid reflux and heartburn disorders.

Baldness and Apple Cider Vinegar

Apple cider vinegar has been offered for its many health benefits. Drinking on a daily basis can help with everything from burning heart to regularity and can also be used topically to help treat a variety of skin diseases, including eczema and warts. One wonders if there is something that apple cider vinegar can not cure. Another thing you will feel is that you can literally look 20 years younger.

Guess what...

For all men (and women) who wish you had the wavy strands of your youth back, it turns out that apple cider vinegar can help. It is also true, although this is not exactly what the old pumice Deleon was looking for, apple cider vinegar can help reverse alopecia and takes ten or two years off the head.

Here's how

Scientists now believe that excessive accumulation of DHT around the radical of the follicle is what causes the death of the hair follicles and becomes unable to produce new hair growth. DHT essentially accumulates around the follicle, like wax, which stifles the blood supply and causes it to shrink and eventually die. Organic apple cider can actually help dissolve this extra build-up of DHT around the follicles and promote the growth of new hair. Acids and enzymes could also help kill some pathogens associated with excess DHT and hair loss due to alopecia.

With help to prevent hair loss, apple cider vinegar also helps to balance the pH of your hair and head, which also helps prevent dandruff and leaves hair healthy and shiny. It also kills all other fungal bacteria that could occur in it.

You will find many natural shampoos and rinse with products that use apple cider vinegar online or in your local grocery store.

Advanced Cosmetics

Keep a 16 oz bottle in the shower. To fill the bottle, pour 1 part vinegar and 3 parts water, then add about 30 drops of essential oils. You can use a mixture of sweet orange, Palmarosa and lavender. It leaves a good smell on your hair and make it really soft. Use only a small amount, leave to act, then rinse. The vial usually takes about 5 days to fill.

Apple Cider Vinegar and Honey Remedy

The health benefits of apple cider vinegar and honey drink are widely known. This recipe has traditionally been used as a personal home remedy for many ailments and even an anti-aging elixir. Many people skillfully used their cleansing and disinfecting properties to self-control their bodies. It is considered as a powerful cleansing agent and natural healing elixir with natural antibiotic and antiseptic that fights germs and bacteria.

Alkalization Diet

So, how does vinegar and honey work? A person's blood circulation, has a tendency to become acidic with our modern diet of fats, starches and processed foods (e.g. fast food, meat, peanuts, seafood, alcohol and coffee) and if your body is acidic, disease can flourish if it is alkaline, it is in balance and can fight germs and diseases, such as bladder and kidney, osteoporosis, brittle bones, joint pain, muscle pain, low energy and chronic fatigue, and slow digestion. Raw fruits, leafy vegetables, legumes and tea are examples of alkaline foods. Interestingly, acid or alkaline tendency of the food in the body has nothing to do with the actual pH of the food itself. For example, lemons and limes are very acidic, but the end products they produce after digestion and assimilation are very alkaline so lemons and limes are alkaline in the body. Likewise, meat will test alkaline before digestion, but leaves the body very acidic residue, so, like nearly all animal products, meat is very acidic. It is important to know that gastric acid or gastric pH is a completely different mass from the pH of fluids and tissues of the body. The body has an acid-alkaline (or acid-base) ratio called the pH which is a balance between positively charged ions (acid formation) and negatively charged ions (alkaline formation). When this balance is disturbed, many problems can arise. The body is forced to borrow minerals - including calcium, sodium, potassium and magnesium from vital organs and bones to neutralize the acid and safely remove it from the body. And serious damage to the body can be caused by high acidity. Ideally, for most people, the ideal diet is 75% alkalizing and 25% acidifying food by volume. Allergic reactions and other forms of stress also tend to produce excess acids in the body.

The alkalinity of apple cider vinegar can correct excessive acidity in our system and help prevent and fight infections. Honey added to vinegar naturally makes the mixture more drinking for people. And the good news is that unprocessed raw honey was classified as an alkaline dish. (Processed honey is little acidifying and artificial sweetener is very acidifying). When you first drink the apple cider vinegar formula, you may taste awful, but as your body becomes less acidic and more alkaline, it would start to taste good. Diseases that can be treated by taking this treatment with apple cider vinegar and honey include:

1. Premature aging

2. Obesity

3. Food poisoning

4. Heat exhaustion

5. Combustion

6. Brittle nails

7. Odor

8. Arthritis

9. Hypertension

10. High cholesterol

Try this healthy and refreshing drink with vinegar and honey! Basically, prepare:

* Mix a tablespoon of apple cider vinegar and a tablespoon of raw honey. (Apple cider vinegar is actually made from fresh, organic, and chopped apples, which can mature naturally in wooden barrels, but you can easily get in the grocery stores or supermarkets.)

* Dissolve in a glass of ice water.

* Take twice a day.

Note: for this vinegar and honey remedy, no commercial distilled vinegars as they do not contain the same health values as the organic raw apple cider vinegar. Powerful enzymes and minerals like potassium, phosphorus, sodium, magnesium, sulfur, copper, iron, fluorine, Silicon, pectin and natural weird and acids, which are important in the fight against toxins from the body and prevent the growth of bacteria, are all destroyed during the distillation process.

10 Reasons to Add Apple Cider Vinegar to Your Diet

Many people have a bottle of apple cider vinegar (ACV) somewhere in the kitchen. Chefs gently add it to enhance the taste of some dishes or as a dressing. They can start using a little more if they know how beneficial this liquid with a sour taste is.

Apple cider vinegar was used as a folk remedy to cure everything from warts to influenza. Even though many claims remain unproven, medical professionals are convinced that adding a touch into your diet can be quite healthy. Experts suggest drinking a teaspoon of apple cider vinegar mixed with water or juice every day. Here are 10 reasons why.

This fluid, which contains acetic acid, has antibiotic properties, which you need when you suffer from diarrhea caused by bacterial infections.

Pectin in apple cider vinegar can help control intestinal spasms and digestive problems.

Does your throat hurt? Gargling infection and bad bacteria with a mixture of a quarter cup of warm water and a quarter cup of special vinegar. Acid kills bacteria.

Scientists believe that after completing animal studies, a newly discovered mixture of acids is also able to lower cholesterol in humans. We need more tests.

Do you often get bored with a stuffy nose or a stuffy nose? Potassium in raw apple cider vinegar can lose weight mucus.

Acetic acid can suppress human appetite, reduce water retention and increase metabolism. Consumption of less calories is equal to weight loss.

Nobody wants dandruff. Mix a quarter cup of water and a quarter cup of this unique type of vinegar in a bottle with a spray. Spray it on your head before you wash your hair. Wrap a towel around your head for 15 minutes. This routine should be done at least twice a week. Your hair will be brighter, too.

Do you need more power? Now you know what to drink to overcome fatigue!

People with eczema problems can cleanse the skin and prevent the epidemic by ingesting apple cider vinegar diluted in water.

Stop poisoning the night leg cramps through the potassium found in apple cider vinegar. Make your new home remedy softer by adding a teaspoon of honey.

Kind reader,

Thank you very much. I hope you enjoyed the book.

Can I ask you a big favor?

I would be grateful if you would please take a few minutes to leave me a gold star on Amazon.

Thank you again for your support.

Anne Duval